The ION Miracle

The effects of negative ions on physical and mental well-being

by

Jean-Yves Côté

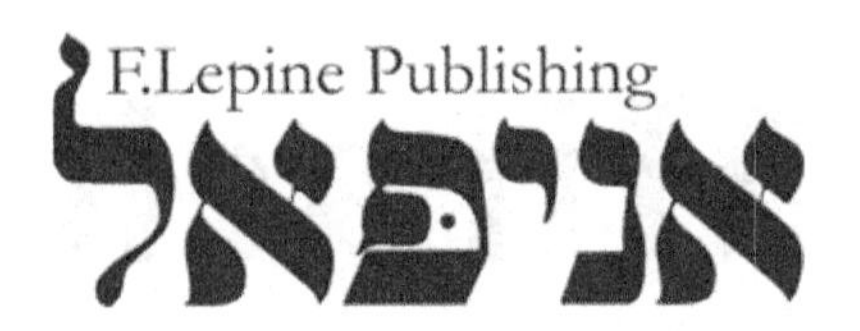

610 des Mélèzes

St-Raymond, Qc G3L 2E9

www.negions.com

ISBN : 978-1-926659-17-6

Illustrations

Violaine Côté

Foreword

On August 1, 1997, I began a contract for a manufacturer of polarized filters and ionizers (negative ion generators). In November, Nicolas Greco, a friend and former biologist, tested an ionizer. “You should look into this further,” he insisted. “I think there is unbelievable potential in this sphere.” Encouraged, I started researching, sifting through the company’s documentation first. John Hurley suggested I read a collection of articles and a small book entitled *The Ion Effect*, by Fred Soyka. The book was a revelation. Unable to find copies of it in Montreal and Toronto, I tried to contact the publisher and author directly. I sent several faxes to Toronto and New York, but without success.

The book was out of print and the author could not be reached. I wanted to have copies made of it for acquaintances, but could not do so without violating copyright law. I continued looking for other books and articles on the subject, but those I found were also out of print. For months, I tried unsuccessfully to contact Dr. Hervé Robert, author of *Ionization, Health Vitality*, and his publisher, Artulen. On a business trip to France, I even consulted the electronic phone book, but neither of the two Hervé Robert's it listed was the author I was looking for.

Finally, convinced of the importance of the subject but unable to find available material about it, I decided to write this book, which both summarizes the literature about and documents personal experiences of the effects of negative ions.

Jean-Yves Côté

Thanks

I am particularly grateful to Nicolas Greco, who urged me to pursue the question of negative ions. Christine Keyser also encouraged me to write this book, saying: "If you can't find any books about ions, write one." Thank you Christine, the work is done. Maïté and Julien Jallet and Robert Cardinal helped me get started, arranging for my use of Christophe Bennegen's apartment during my stay in Bois D' Arcy, France. The first pages were difficult, but I had to start somewhere. My thanks to Estelle Poudrette and my daughter Héloise, who helped me gather my notes in the form of a book. Thanks also to my daughter Violaine for her illustrations and photographs. Finally, I want to express my gratitude to Francine Quirion, my companion, for her support and encouragement in bringing this book into being.

Table of Contents

Chapter 1

Fred Soyka's Experience

Mr. Soyka worked in New York for an American multi-national corporation. In 1961, he accepted a transfer to Geneva, where he lived for eight years. Except for a persistent bad cold, the first year of his stay was enjoyable. In the second year, the cold worsened, and he began suffering stomach and headaches as well. He felt nauseous after meals, tried to avoid social gatherings and experienced diminished sex drive. Finally, he felt so unwell that he decided to see a doctor. He had poor digestion and felt run down, out of shape, anxious and stressed. His doctor referred him to a gastroenterologist, who diagnosed a malfunctioning gall bladder and prescribed its removal.

Before the surgery, Soyka went on a two-week trip to New York. By the second day, the symptoms that had troubled him in Geneva had disappeared. He felt great. On one occasion, he ate fast food and digested it without difficulty. Back in Geneva, he called his specialist and told him that his gall bladder had functioned perfectly in New York and that the diagnosis was wrong.

Within two weeks, however, all his symptoms had returned. His doctor sent him to another specialist, who told him that, like many other people in Geneva, he was suffering hypothyroidism. The specialist prescribed stimulants for his thyroid, and a few days later Soyka felt much better. He was now taking tranquilizers to calm his nerves during periods of anxiety and stimulants to shake his feeling of apathy. Sometimes he took sleeping pills. He began to depend on pills the way other people depend on alcohol.

In 1964, Soyka became vice-president of his company, but his health problems persisted. Most of the time, he felt well and full of energy. But on some days, without apparent reason, he felt tense and anxious, unable to function normally. These periods were marked by insomnia and followed by moments of hyperactivity or total lassitude and paralyzing despair. The simplest tasks, such as making a phone call or putting out the garbage, seemed overwhelming.

A strange fact had escaped Soyka's attention. Whenever he left Geneva on business trips or family vacations, his appetite returned. He could have digested nails without heartburn. His mood and energy level recovered too. Stranger yet, these recoveries occurred even when his travels took him elsewhere within Europe.

In 1965, his doctor suggested that his disorders were psychosomatic. For the next two years, Soyka spent four hours a week consulting a psychiatrist, who examined such issues as his irrational fears and his real or supposed guilt. In the past, Soyka had scorned psychiatric help, seeing it as a sign of weakness and of an unwillingness to solve personal problems. Now, on the brink of suicide, he agreed to therapy. But after two years of psychiatric care, his health had not improved. He wrote in his diary: "Very ill, depressed, feel discouraged," " Sleepless night again! Felt like the dead, and wish I were." He worried about everything, and even worried about worry itself.

During his eighth year in Geneva, in spite of professional success, he again felt bad enough to consult a doctor, turning this time to Dr. Wissmer, a physician with many foreign patients. Wissmer told him that many of his patients suffered from similar symptoms: colds, tiredness, poor digestion, depression, diminished sex drive. Wissmer believed this phenomenon was related to the electricity in the air in Geneva. The majority of his patients not only suffered from the same ills as Soyka, but also experienced similar bouts of irrational behavior. The divorce rate among foreigners, for example, was abnormally high. The men complained that their spouses or partners no longer excited them, when in fact they were experiencing diminished sex drive. Some embarked on new adventures or short-lived sexual frenzies, only to return to their former listlessness. The women complained that they felt anxious and unhappy, and blamed their distress on a lack of interest in sex. Wissmer had also noted other problems that were common to foreigners, such as immoderate alcohol consumption and tension. The Swedish wife of a businessman had caught a cold on her arrival in Geneva and continued to have it for the next ten years. She often felt she had changed: she yelled at the children, criticized her husband, ate too much and became increasingly overweight. She became so depressed and ill tempered that she couldn't stand herself. Before arriving in Geneva, this woman had lived happily in several European and Middle-Eastern countries.

Wissmer had noticed that patients who suffered Soyka's symptoms all seemed to visit him at the same time. His practice would operate at a normal pace for a while, until suddenly and without warning, all his foreign patients would call in on the same day.

Chapter two

Winds that kill

"You shall not judge when the Sharav blows."

Talmud

"It is the very error of the moon;
She comes more nearer earth than she was wont,
And makes men mad."

Shakespeare, *Othello*

Soyka's symptoms are shared by many people who live in areas of the world that experience dry winds, called witches' winds in several languages. These symptoms also occur during the full moon and before storms. Popular expressions record our sensitivity to atmospheric conditions: when we're unwell, we feel "under the weather;" before a storm approaches, we "feel it in our bones." Hippocrates, the father of modern medicine, had also noticed a correlation between temperature and certain diseases.

The lines quoted from the Talmud at the beginning of the chapter were probably written in Israel, where a desert wind blows that is called the Sharav in Hebrew and the Khamsin in Arabic. It is one of a number of witches' winds, of which the following are the most familiar:

Switzerland, Germany, Tyrol	Foehn
Toulouse region, France	Vent d'Autan
Provence and Côte d'Azur, France	Mistral
California, USA	Santa Ana
Italy	Sirocco
Argentina	Zonda
Rockies, Canada	Chinook
Egypt	Sharkije
Spain	Lévante
India	Thor
Australia	Northern Wind
Middle-East	Sharav or Khamsin

One day, Soyka called Helen Eliat van de Velde, a psychologist who had studied throughout Europe before settling in New York. She had noticed that on certain days, the majority of her patients felt optimistic and enthusiastic, while on others, the majority felt depressed and unhappy. She had kept note of the temperature, but could find no correlation between the weather and her clients' mood swings. While Soyka was with her, her phone rang constantly. She told him that her patients all experienced crises at the same time. Earlier in the day, a patient had spit blood from a ruptured stomach ulcer. At lunch, van de Velde was interrupted by a patient, a beautiful model in her twenties, who said that she felt unable to face the cameras that day. A violinist couldn't play because his hands were trembling and clammy. "A hurricane is blowing in from the Caribbean," the psychologist said, opening the window. "I know the sun is shining and it's a beautiful day, but come listen." From outside, Soyka heard the voices of angry taxi drivers, arguing over the sound of the traffic. " I tell you, my patients and the taxi drivers are barometers. My patients are more prone to problems and the taxi drivers get more aggressive whenever the weather is about to change (Soyka 12)." That night, the temperature changed and

Soyka slept badly, experiencing the symptoms he had suffered in Geneva. In the morning, the newspapers reported that a storm had changed its course in the Caribbean and threatened the southern states.

The Swiss blame many unusual occurrences on the Foehn: suicides, murders, car accidents, domestic disputes. Surgeons in the Munich area postpone surgeries when the Foehn is forecast.

Soyka had a friend in Munich who occasionally suffered from insomnia. During those sleepless nights, she would hear the whistles of trains passing in the distance. The sound was carried from the south by the Foehn. Another of his friends felt literally suffocated whenever the Foehn blew. To find relief, she would walk along a bridge at the foot of a waterfall. Looking at her, one might have thought she was a fascinated passer-by, enjoying the view of the bubbling water; in fact, she was there to catch her breath. Half an hour by the falls would ease her breathing for several hours to come.

One may wonder what the moon, the witches' winds and oncoming storms all have in common, other than the effect they have on people.

Since its discovery by Benjamin Franklin, researchers have shown that electricity affects plant and animal life. In 1775, Father Giambattista Becceria of the university at Turin wrote: "Nature makes great use of atmospheric electricity to develop vegetation (Métadier 9)." During the 19th century, various researchers studied the influence of electricity on plant growth. In 1899, Elster and Geitel discovered the existence of ions, but the systematic study of the effects of ions on life only began three decades later.

In 1930, Hansell, an American researcher, observed that a laboratory assistant who worked next to an electrostatic generator experienced mood swings when the generator changed polarity. When the polarity of the generator was negative, he felt euphoric and full of energy. When the polarity was positive, however, his mood darkened and he felt depressed and aggressive.

Extensive research has since been conducted to investigate electric polarity in the air. In the 1970's, Soyka could already count more than 5000 related projects, studies and experiments. Almost all concluded that negatively charged ions enhance our well-being, while positively charged ions are harmful to us.

As we know, atoms consist of a positively-charged core surrounded by negatively-charged electrons. Because the electrons and the core carry an equal charge, atoms are neutral. When electrons are freed from the core, however, the atom becomes positive and is called a positive ion or pos-ion. If, on the other hand, the neutral atom captures an electron, it is negatively charged, and is called a negative ion or neg-ion. If this positive or negative atom (positive ion or negative ion) is incorporated in a molecule, the molecule becomes an ion, and if this ion is fixed in a group of molecules, such as soot, dust, or liquid droplets, they also become positive or negative ions. Following standard usage, any small particle carrying an electric charge will be referred to as an ion throughout this book.

In nature, the usual ion ratio is 12 pos-ions for 10 neg-ions. But these proportions vary enormously from place to place according to barometric pressure, prevailing winds, the radioactivity of the ground and pollution. Places that have high concentrations of neg-ions, such as sea shores, mountains, rivers and waterfalls, attract us when we want to enjoy rest and relaxation. Before an electrical storm, when the atmosphere is heavy, it is charged with pos-ions. After the storm, the air feels invigorating and we often breathe deeply to enjoy its sweetness. At this time, the air is highly charged with neg-ions. During rush hour, city air is almost completely depleted of neg-ions. Because of the so-called Faraday Cage Effect, the air in cars is also poor in neg-ions. We will discuss each of these points farther on.

Soyka met a young Montreal couple at the start of their honeymoon on the Riviera. They were quite unhappy. The groom, a young lawyer, as enthusiastic as one would expect on such an occasion, suddenly began arguing with his wife on the day after their arrival. He felt acutely tense, and then extremely tired. The Mistral, the witches' winds of southern France, was blowing. A few days later, the couple moved on to continue their honeymoon under other, less romantic skies. The husband's good mood returned and the honeymoon ended pleasantly. Winston Churchill chose the dates of his trips to the southern coast of France carefully, in order to avoid the season of the Mistral.

On the West Coast of Canada and the United States, the Chinook blows down from the mountains at the beginning of spring. Although it is a welcome harbinger of spring, doctors report an increase in colds and other respiratory problems during this period. Soyka knew an industrialist who lived in this area. For ten years, he not only suffered the usual seasonal colds, but also felt anxious and tense when the Chinook blew. He learned to plan vacation trips in spring, in order to avoid the windy period.

The Santa Ana, the witches' winds of California, blows from Hollywood and Los Angeles down to San Diego. The belief that the Santa Ana causes violence, murders and suicides is so widespread that screenwriters developed a police show in which the wind is responsible for the crimes committed by the characters.

Besides the Foehn, the Sharav or Khamsin is undoubtedly the most studied of the witches' winds, due in large part to the work of Dr. Sulman of the University of Jerusalem. Sulman studied the effects of the Sharav on human behavior. He began by collecting anecdotal evidence of these effects. A shoemaker showed him sales figures that were 300% higher during Sharav, when people found that their feet swelled and they needed larger shoes. Psychiatrists told him that their patients tended to be more distressed than usual at these times. An insurance salesman claimed that the accident rate increased by 100%, and the police reported that acts of aggression such as domestic violence also rose during Sharav. Military officers said that soldiers stationed on desert frontiers for long periods of time became lethargic and depressed. In some translations of the book of Isaiah, the Sharav is described as "bad" and "destructive".

During earlier research in the field of gynecology, Sulman had shown that serotonin influences the human body and emotions. He went on to conduct a four-year study to determine the serotonin level in healthy subjects who were not sensitive to the Sharav. He selected subjects from his personnel.

Daily urine tests were taken to measure how much serotonin is manufactured by the body and how much of it is transformed into in an inoffensive substance commonly referred to as 5HA. The study concluded that serotonin is only present in the urine of healthy human subjects when they are anxious or under great emotional stress.

We have long known that the body produces adrenaline in response to known stressors that are usually external, such as aggression or the writing of an exam. While adrenaline is produced in response to dangers perceived by the five senses, serotonin seems to be excreted in response to dangers that are imperceptible to the senses. For example, emotional stress and anxiety seem to produce serotonin.

After this study, Sulman began testing Sharav victims. In little time he had recruited more than 200 volunteers. They were men and women, young and old, of all social classes and from various countries, all so affected by Sharav that they were ready to participate as test subjects in the hope of finding relief. For a year, the volunteers had to come in twice every day to submit urine samples for analysis. The study concluded that these people produced 1000% more serotonin during Sharav, while their ability to break down serotonin into the inoffensive 5HA only doubled, leaving a significant serotonin surplus in their bodies. But how could the wind produce such effects?

In the 1950s and 1960s, Krueger, an American researcher, established a link between the production of serotonin and the presence of pos-ions. On the basis of Krueger's theory, Sulman recruited physicists and meteorologists to measure the electrical nature of the Sharav. On days when the Sharav doesn't blow, the ion count in Jerusalem is generally between 1,000 and 2,000 positive and negative ions per cubic centimeter. Two days before the Sharav, the quantity of ions per cubic centimeter doubles and the proportion of pos-ions increases considerably. The conclusion was obvious: the only variable that could explain the abnormal production of serotonin in people sensitive to the Sharav was the very great concentration of pos-ions in the air during the wind's passage.

Dr. Rehn, a German surgeon, practiced in a hospital in Freiburg, near Munich, where the cases of postoperative hemorrages were especially frequent during Foehn weather. He later moved to Ettenheim, 40 kilometers from Freiburg. There, citizens were protesting against a factory that produced red clouds of smoke. Rehn noted that the hospital reported no cases of thrombosis. The government obliged the factory to clean up its emissions, and the red cloud disappeared. At the same time, the rates of hemorrhage increased, matching those of Freiburg. Interestingly, a doctor named Spitzer had measured the air electricity prior to the change and had noted a very high concentration of neg-ions. After the disappearance of the polluting cloud, Ettenheim also experienced the effects of the Foehn, like other cities in the area.

The so-called witches' winds that we have described above are all charged with pos-ions. The negative effects attributed to these winds can be explained by the fact that they are over-charged with pos-ions and almost depleted of neg-ions. The witches' winds originate in the high atmosphere. As they approach the earth, they come into contact with other masses. The resulting friction seems to destroy neg-ions. Some of these winds, such as the Sharav, travel over dry land where they lift a lot of dust. Neg-ions, which are primarily small oxygen ions, combine easily with dust and are soon entirely absorbed, leaving only pos-ions in the wind. The fact that the neg-ions have been leeched from the air because they have attached themselves to dust and moisture may explain the discomfort felt in cities and prior to storms when the air is humid. Storms break when the atmosphere is saturated and heavily charged with pos-ions. Since the earth is negatively charged, it attracts these positive charges. Lighting and rain rid the atmosphere of pos-ions and create an overproduction of neg-ions, leaving the air fresh and invigorating. The same phenomena occur alongside waterfalls and rivers and by the seashore, especially when the surf is up. As water droplets move through the air, they cast off a fine spray that is charged with neg-ions. Since learning this, I have thought that having a water fountain near one's home is a precious asset.

Effects similar to those produced by the witches' winds have been recorded prior to storms and during the full moon. Soyka documents interesting events that seem to be related to the lunar cycle (p. 60-61). Dr. Shealy, a neurosurgeon and director of the Pain Clinic at La Crosse, Wisconsin, questioned his colleagues and discovered that severe hemorrhages are most common when the moon is full. He also studied data from blood banks, discovering that the demand for blood transfusions

is consistently higher during the full moon and the few days which follow.
At the Tallahassee Hospital in Florida, Dr. Edson Andrew kept statistics about some 1,000 patients he had operated on, and noted that 82% of serious postoperative hemorrhages occured when the moon is full.

A few years ago, I met a telephone operator who handled international calls. She told me that during the time of the full moon, there were many more requests for long-distance calls and that people often behaved irrationally, making incoherent remarks and speaking rudely. For her, full-moon evenings were a terrible strain.

Dr. Sulman wanted to understand what causes repeated miscarriages. He assumed that women who repeatedly miscarry produce too much serotonin. He initially experimented on pregnant rats, which invariably aborted after being injected with serotonin. Afterwards, he conducted a study with 20 women who wanted to abort and had received their physicians' consent to do so. These women were given drugs that stimulate the body to produce an overdose of serotonin. In all cases, the patients aborted. He continued his investigation with women who had suffered repeated miscarriages and discovered high levels of serotonin in their urine. He proposed treatments that also sensitized husbands to the situation, involving them in practical details such as urine collection. When the women felt less pressured and anxious, their serotonin levels dropped. Drugs that inhibit the production of serotonin made it possible for many of these women to give birth to normal, healthy children. This, like other studies reported above, suggests that people sensitive to pos-ions produce a high quantity of serotonin. Sulman estimates that approximately 30% of the population is affected by temperature changes, witches' winds and the full moon, all of which create high concentrations of pos-ions. The fact that more children are born when the moon is full may be due to the abundance of pos-ions in the air during this period. In its full phase, the moon puts pressure on the ionosphere (which begins approximately 40 kilometers above ground). Because the ground is negatively charged, the pos-ions in the ionosphere are drawn to the ground, passing through our atmosphere and accumulating more intense positive charges on the way.

Reliable equipment is now available to measure the quantity of ions in a given environment. Whatever theories researchers propose to explain the presence or absence of ions, we now know with certainty that positive and negative ions exist, and we are able to measure their concentrations and recognize their effects on human behavior and health. These discoveries are all the more important because we live and work in artificial environments that are depleted of neg-ions and thus detrimental to our well being and health. Fortunately, we are able to recognize the problem. In many cases, we can also resolve it by eliminating the sources of pos-ion production and creating neg-ion generators, such as water fountains and ionizers.

Chapter 3

Sanctuaries of life

Throughout the world, people vacation in places that have the highest concentrations of positive ions. Perhaps we have an innate wisdom or ability to recognize what is good for us.

Nature produces witches' winds charged with pos-ions, but it also offers spaces where high concentrations of neg-ions create sanctuaries of life. There are many natural sources of neg-ion production. In the lower atmosphere, the most important is the natural radioactivity of rocks. When the radioactive gases produced by rocks enters the air, their radiation produces ion pairs. However, because the mass of the earth is negative, pos-ions tend to be magnetically drawn towards the ground, leaving the air charged with neg-ions. This may explain why mountain air seems so refreshing.

Perhaps it also explains the legendary longevity of people who live in mountainous regions.

Another very important source of neg-ions is chlorophyllous photosynthesis, the production of oxygen by chlorophyll exposed to daylight. We have long known that plants create oxygen, but we now know also that the oxygen that is produced is negatively charged. This explains why country and forest air seems so rich to city dwellers, and also underscores the importance of parks in urban areas.

We feel exhilarated by quick-running water, experience bliss at the foot of waterfalls, and feel invigorated by the smell of waves breaking on rocks. We appreciate fountains in our parks and cities. We get relief from a good shower after a day at work, a ride in the car or a tense meeting. All these places are negatively charged because of the so-called Lénard effect, whereby neg-ions are produced by the friction of water droplets breaking up in the air.

In the 18th century, Saussure observed that people who live by waterfalls live healthier, longer lives. Thermal springs have always offered relief to people who suffer from respiratory problems or tension. Previously, their benefits were attributed to the quality of their water, but it is likely that the oveproduction of neg-ions by fountains and pools also contributes to their effects.

The friction of air moving against sharp-pointed solids produces neg-ions. Because of their millions of needles, pine forests generate an overproduction of neg-ions, especially on windy days. This explains why health centers that offer both thermal springs and pine forests can be so beneficial. Perhaps this is also why the cedars of Lebanon have always symbolized beauty and happiness.

Chapter 4

Research and experiments

In the following pages, we will summarize the results of studies reported by F. Soyka, J. Métadier and H. Robert in the books listed in the bibliography. The findings are discussed by topic. For the sake of brevity, we will not always signal the source, which is generally one of the authors named above. In some instances, the same studies are mentioned by all three.

As mentioned earlier, interest in air electricity goes back a few hundreds years. Systematic research began in the 1930s, but was brought to a halt by the Second World War. After the war, it was resumed primarily in Russia, where researchers were particularly interested in the influence of neg-ions on the development of athletes and in the treatment of certain respiratory diseases.

No ions, no life

In Russia, Tchijewsky tried raising small animals in a well-oxygenated atmosphere that contained no ions. After a few days, they all died. Tchijewsky concluded that we need ions to absorb enough oxygen to survive. Dr. Krueger showed that endurance, health and well-being improve in the presence of a strong concentration of neg-ions.

Ions for athletes

After the Second World War, a Russian researcher named A. A. Minkh conducted a series of experiments with high-performance athletes. Forty athletes were required to lift 3-5 kg weights at a rate of one lift per second. When the test subjects were exhausted, one group received overdoses of neg-ions, a second received overdoses of both positive and negative ions and a third group was left to recover in the surrounding air. The group which had received an overdose of neg-ions recovered first, followed by those who had received a combined overdose of positive and negative ions, while those left untreated recovered last. The study concluded that athletes recover more quickly in the presence of neg-ions.

In another experiment, athletes were asked to run on the spot at a rate of 180 steps/minute until exhaustion. One group trained in an atmosphere enriched with neg-ions, the other in untreated ambient air. Initially, the two groups turned in comparable performances. After one month, however, the group exposed to neg-ions had increased its endurance by 240%. This level remained high over the next ten days without additional neg-ions, and then stabilized at 38%. The endurance of the control group also improved, but only from 7 to 24%, and their endurance level fell off more quickly than that of the neg-ion group.

Reaction time to visual stimuli was also measured. The variations are slight, but for an Olympic athlete, a few milliseconds can make the difference between a gold medal and no medal at all. Carroll measured the reaction time of athletes to the sound signals that mark the start of a race. After three hours of negative ionization, the athletes' average reaction time dropped from 72 to 65 milliseconds, a 10% improvement.

Hawkins measured reaction time to visual and sound stimuli, noting that visual response ranged from 188 milliseconds in normal air, to 165 in positively- and 158 in negatively-ionized air. Buchalew used dynamometers to measure handgrip: subjects in the control group obtained a result of 555, while those in neg-ion enriched air registered 666.

Good for plants, lethal for bacteria

The first studies of the effects of air electricity involved plants. As early as 1748, Nollet, a priest, had observed an acceleration in growth rates when a charged electrode was placed over plants. All subsequent studies have confirmed that plant growth is optimized by the presence of strong concentrations of positive or negative ions.

Studies carried out by Elkiey on barley cultivated in an atmosphere enriched by 400,000 neg-ions per cubic centimeter indicated a 15% growth increase, and an 18% increase in dry weight.

In a greenhouse equipped with neg-ion generators, not only did plants grow more quickly, but insects and molds disappeared at such a rate that the pesticide program could be stopped (Métadier 131). Bacteria and other micro-organisms are destroyed by high concentrations of neg-ions.

The first discoveries made by Dr. Krueger, an American celebrity in the field of air ion research, concluded that the presence of neg-ions in the air, even in small quantities, destroys airborne bacteria which are the primary sources of transmission of respiratory illnesses such as colds and influenza.

Professor Krauss, of the Institute of Hygiene of the University of Hanover in Germany, noted an 87% reduction of bacteria in a room ionized for one hour, and a 97% reduction after 100 minutes.

Dr. Kellog studied the survival rate of the gilded staphylococcus, the germ most often responsible for cutaneous infections. Germs in a concentration of one million parts per ml were placed in a bottle. After five hours in a non-ionized atmosphere, the concentration contained one million fifty parts per ml, and the ionized air was completely free of germs.

Estula studied viral transmission among chickens. Chickens were given 0.3 ml of a solution containing 100 million Newcastle virus per ml, and then placed among other chickens. All the inoculated animals died. In normal air, 75% of chickens placed alongside the inoculated birds also died; in ionized air, there was no contamination, and all the non-inoculated chickens survived.

One of the conclusions of these studies is that both kinds of ions have a bactericidal effect. Pos-ions, however, have only an electrical effect, whereas neg-ions also have a chemico-biological effect that is lethal to bacteria. The microbicidal effect of neg-ions may be due to the fact that the majority of neg-ions are oxygen ions and oxygen destroys microbes.

Camille Ringuette, my business partner, offered an ionizer to her sister Andrée. Andrée had leukemia and required regular chemotherapy treatments. After every treatment, she suffered weeks of fever and infections.

One of the effects of chemotherapy is that it shuts down the immune system. After installing the ionizer in her room, however, Andrée no longer developed fevers or infections after her treatments. Her doctor was astonished.

The nurse who treated Andrée said she had never seen anything comparable in six years of work with cancer patients. In October 1998, Andrée received a bone marrow transplant. When she visited me some seventy days after the operation, she said that no other patient at the hospital had ever recovered from a bone marrow transplant without fever or infection. Did the ionizer help strengthen Andrée's immune system, encourage relaxation or eliminate bacteria and viruses in her immediate environment? Whatever the answer, Andrée blesses her sister for having given her such a precious gift.

Animal research

After five weeks in an ionized atmosphere, turkeys increase in weight by 5%, despite a 4% drop in food consumption. Seven weeks later, relative weight gain remains at 5%, but food consumption drops by another 8%. After 26 days of negative ionization, rabbits experience a 20% weight increase; after 14 days, pigs show a 23% increase. While this is good news for stockbreeders, it may worry people who are concerned about weight loss. Stress is considered to be an important factor in bulimia and anorexia. The relaxation induced by neg-ions should help correct compulsive eating disorders and regulate behavior.

Given a choice of three cages, one with pos-ions, one with ambient air and one with neg-ions, mice never choose the positively ionized cage. While a few mice enter the ambient air cage, most throng into the cage enriched with neg-ions.

American researchers succeeded in making rabbits, which are the most peaceful of domestic animals, aggressive by exposing them to overdoses of pos-ions.

In another American experiment, young and old rats were placed in a labyrinth. In normal air, the young rats escaped from the labyrinth more quickly than the old. In air enriched with neg-ions, the old rats performed as well as the young.

An experiment using T-mazes also concluded that neg-ions rejuvenate the mind. In normal air, old rats made three times more mistakes than young rats. In negatively ionized air, the old rats performed as accurately and as quickly as the young.

Burn victims of Philadelphia

In 1958, Dr. Igho Kornblueh, of General Northeastern Hospital at Philadelphia, undertook a systematic study of 187 patients suffering from burns of various degree. He treated a control group of 49 people with standard medication. The 138 others were treated with the neg-ions. Only 59 of the latter group experienced no improvement. The 79 others felt pain relief and healed more quickly. While 57.3% of patients treated with ions showed improvement, only 22.5% of the control group experienced comparable recovery. Astonished by the spectacular results, the researchers involved in the study were unwilling to draw conclusions. Dr. Minehart, who had played an important role in setting up the experiment, was incredulous: "At first I thought that it was voodoo, now I'm convinced that it is real and revolutionary" (Soyka 65). The results were so convincing that the hospital equipped all its post-operative rooms with ionizers. In 1971, Soyka visited Dr. Kornblueh in

Philadelphia. The physician was embittered. Although the Philadelphia research was conclusive, no other hospital had adopted ion therapy. He understood that people might be cautious, but was enraged at the thought of the preventable pain, unnecessary drug treatment and slow recovery which burn victims were left to suffer because of the failure of medical authorities to act on the findings of ion therapy research.

The Philadelphia study noted that, when treated with negative ions, burn victims who also had bronchitis or asthma experienced simultaneous relief of their respiratory problems. Encouraged by these results, Kornblueh undertook another series of experiments, this time at the teaching hospital of the University of Pennsylvania and with people suffering from respiratory illnesses. 63% of the treated patients experienced partial or complete recovery. These results led Kornblueh to describe neg-ions as "vitamins of the air".

Soyka records another example involving burn treatment. A British television host received second-degree burns when she accidentally scalded her chest with hot tea. She treated herself with an ionizer she had bought to counter a mild case of asthma, holding the neg-ion generator against her wound three times a day. After two days, the pain subsided and the wounds started to heal. Two weeks later, the burn had healed without leaving a trace. She was thrilled, delighted to think that she would be able to wear a bikini again.

Respiratory problems

Throughout the world, the incidence of respiratory illnesses is on the rise. In the United States alone, it is estimated that over 30 million people suffer from some form of respiratory illness or allergies involving the respiratory system, such as allergies to pollen, dust or cigarette smoke. Over the last decade, the number of cases has increased by 80%

among women, 50% among children and 30% among men. Given that the air inside modern buildings is considered to be four times more polluted than that outside, the fact that women and children spend more time indoors may explain these numbers. In order to save money and energy, we recirculate air that has been treated by heating or cooling systems. Indoor air is also poisoned by the dust of the detergents and chemicals we use. Particles smaller than 10 microns remain suspended in the air indefinitely; detergents produce a fine dust that is between .05 and 5 microns in size, and thus accumulates easily.

By 1975, a German doctor had already used neg-ion therapy to treat more than 11,000 patients suffering respiratory. He said that his patients reported back to him with monotonous regularity to confirm the efficacy of the treatment.

A professor living in Thunderbridge Wells in the south of London became allergic to dust after the birth of her first child. She was soon so handicapped that she was unable to do housework. Even cooking had become unpleasant because flour dust provoked all her symptoms: violent headaches, nasal drip and shortness of breath. Her husband, who worked in electronics, bought her an ionizer. She would sit beside it and feel an almost instantaneous effect, as though she had been touched by a magic wand (Soyka 74). The ionizer gave her such complete relief that she could put her apron back on and resume her tasks.

My sister Monique, who lives in Quebec, had a similar though less prolonged experience. She had started an accounting contract with a new company. After a while, she developed a sinusitis accompanied by constant nasal drip. None of the drugs she tried provided relief. On one of my visits to Quebec, my mother told me about my sister's difficulties. Initially I paid no attention, but when she repeated her account one month later, I called my sister to inquire. Monique said that the carpeting at work was old and might be the cause of her problems. Her boss intended to buy her an air purifier. I suggested that he buy an ionizer instead. He did, and the ionizer was installed the following Monday. By midday, Monique's allergies had disappeared.

Nicolas Greco, who represents in Morocc a company that manufactures ionizers, wanted to open the market by approaching physicians. He spoke about his plans with a friend, a doctor in Casablanca, and let him test an ionizer for a few days. Two days later, Greco received a call. The physician, father of an asthmatic girl, had placed the ionizer in his daughter's bedroom. Since its installation, the girl hadn't coughed, and for the first time in years, she had slept through the night.

Richard Rhéaume is from Quebec and sells ionizers in Norway. One Christmas, he gave his parents an ionizer, which they placed in their bedroom. His niece, an asthmatic, spent the night in her grandparents' room. She slept quietly, untroubled by the coughing spells that disturbed her sleep at home.

According to Hervé Robert, the effect of neg-ions on pulmonary allergies can be explained as follows. (Robert, p. 133) The respiratory tract is lined with tiny filaments bathed in mucus. Normally, these filaments, or cilia, vibrate at a rate of 800 beats a minute; pos-ions cause the rate of vibration to drop to 200 beats a minute, and also inhibit mucus production. As a result, dust that enters the respiratory system cannot be cleared out, causing the symptoms that are typical of pulmonary ailments. Perhaps this explains why in past generations, men who lived in the countryside were able to smoke all their lives without developing lung problems. Because their environment was healthy, the cilia in their respiratory tract worked effectively, bringing up smoke dust during the night. In a positively charged environment, on the other hand, the cilia stiffen, inhibiting the body's ability to clean out dust.

Pollen has always been present in the human environment. Why has there recently been such a dramatic increase in the number of people allergic to pollen? Again, the presence of pos-ions may offer an explanation. Slowed by pos-ions, the cilia cannot do their work adequately. When exposed to high doses of neg-ions, however, the cilia recover and mucus production resumes. Because the cause of the allergies is eliminated, the symptoms disappear too.

Neg-ions and sex

We spoke earlier of Soyka's diminished sex drive during Foehn conditions in Geneva. In his book, he tells of other interesting cases. Soyka once asked a sales manager, a quiet, peaceful and rather silent man, if he had noticed any changes since the installation of table ionizers in all the company's offices. To Soyka's surprise, the man answered, "Well, the biggest effect has been on my sex life. My wife loves it" (Soyka 124). The ionizer in his office had made him feel revitalized, and so he had decided to buy one for his car, too, given the many hours he spent driving. He had also put one in his bedroom. In the past, he would return home exhausted, with only enough strength to eat and watch television. Now he felt more energetic. He and his wife had started going out again, and in bed he felt energetic, too. His sex life and marriage had improved significantly.

A bull in a negatively-charged environment shows improved sperm quality. After four days of treatment with neg-ions, male mice exhibit testicular over-activity (Métadier 60) and increased sperm production. In female mice, neg-ions stimulate the ovaries and help regulate the menstrual cycle. In several Eastern European countries, birthing rooms are ionized and neg-ion treatment is given to mothers who have difficulty nursing their newborns. Neg-ion treatment for lactation has proven to be effective for women who have difficulty producing milk, but it seems to have no effect on women who have a normal milk supply.

Rheumatism

In Russia, acute rheumatoid arthritis has been treated with neg-ion therapy since the 1940's. Tchijevshi reports that after 10 sessions, the full recovery rate was 20%; after 25 sessions, the rate of clear improvement was 40%, with 28% of cases showing average improvement, 10% no improvement and 2% a worsening of symptoms (Robert 128).

Figurovky notes that neg-ion therapy alleviates pain in 80% of osteoarthritis attacks.

Teaching problem children

The effect of neg-ions on attention and learning has also been studied. All the research in this area shows that neg-ions counter-act fatigue and enhance concentration and reaction time. The studies also show that the results of neg-ion therapy are particularly impressive in stressful environments, with anxious subjects and with problem children (Robert 167). Of all the people affected by pos-ions, problem children benefit most from exposure to an atmosphere rich in neg-ions.

Researchers and doctors have developed neg-ion treatments for a wide range of diseases. Robert's presentation of this work is particularly interesting. The health benefits of neg-ions are too numerous to discuss here in detail, and are summarized instead in the following table. The information is drawn primarily from Appendix I of Robert's book, and Appendices I and II of Métadier's.

Table: The effects of neg-ions

1	**General**	
1.2	Physical performance	Improved
1.3	Endurance	Increased
1.4	Mood	Positive
1.5	Reaction time	Improved
1.6	Vitamin metabolism	Improved
1.7	Pain	Relieved
1.8	Alertness (drivers in particular)	Improved
1.9	Allergies	Relieved
1.10	Burn treatment	Improved
1.11	Cicatrization	Accelerated
1.12	Sleep	Improved
1.13	Sex drive	Improved
1.14	Fatigue	Reduced
1.15	Vitality	Improved
1.16	Recovery time	Faster

2	**Respiratory system**	
2.1	Adverse effects	none
2.2	Bronchial spasms	Suppressed
2.3	Bronchial permeability	Improved
2.4	Respiratory rate	Decreased
2.5	Partial pressure, oxygen	Increased
2.6	Partial pressure, CO_2	Decreased
2.7	Congestion of the respiratory system	Alleviated
2.8	Asthma	56% recovery, 34% improvement
2.9	Tachypnea	Decreased
2.10	Inflammation of the respiratory tracts	Decreased

3	**Heart**	
3.1	Tension	Regularized
3.2	Thrombosis	Risk reduced
3.3	Heart rate	Slowed down

4	**Brain**	
4.1	Serotonin (Anxiety, aggressiveness or depression)	Decreased
4.2	Alpha waves	-Reduced frequency -Increased amplitude

5	**Endocrine glands**	
5.1	Hypothalamus	Increased secretions
5.2	Pituitary gland	Increased secretions
5.3	Thyroid	Increased secretions
5.4	Suprarenal	Cortisol increases
5.5	Ovaries	-improved ovulation -menstrual cycle regularized
5.6	Testicles	Sperm improved

6	**Rheumatism**	
6.1	Pain	Decreased
6.2	Sedimentation test	Decreased
6.3	Osteoarthritis attacks	Decreased
6.4	Cortisol	Increased
7	**Stomach**	
7.1	Gastric acidity	Decreased
7.2	Risk of hemorrhage	Decreased
7.3	Ulcers	Less frequent

8	**Blood**	
8.1	Cholesterol	Lowered
8.2	Serotonin	Lowered
8.3	Glucose	Lowered
8.4	Vitamins	Increased
8.5	Hemoglobin	Better oxygenation
8.6	Acidity	Lowered
8.7	Sedimentation test	Lowered
8.8	Viscosity	Lowered
8.9	Immune system	Stimulated

9	**Urine**	
9.1	Serotonin	Lowered
9.2	Potassium	Increased
9.3	Diuresis	Increased

10	**Skin**	
10.1	Wounds, burns	Healed
10.2	Skin diseases	Improved
10.3	Hair loss	Decreased
10.4	**Allergies**	
10.5	Anaphylactic shock	Protection
10.6	Rhinitis	Improved
10.7	Asthma	Improved
11	**Mental**	
11.1	Learning	Improved, especially in problem children and the elderly
11.2	Anxiety	Decreased
11.3	Anguish	Decreased
11.4	Depression	Improvement
11.5	Stress	Better control

Chapter 5

Our modern environment: a pos-ion generator

The natural phenomena that produce pos-ions are momentary, transitory. The full moon doesn't shine every night; witches' winds do not blow continuously; storms do not always loom on the horizon. But in our modern world, we have created an environment that is permanently charged with pos-ions or sapped of neg-ions. Generally, there are some 6,000 particles suspended in every milliliter of country air, while city air contains several million particles per milliliter. Perhaps this unfavorable environment is the source of some of the social problems that we see: violence, depression, suicide, anxiety, allergies, pulmonary diseases, cancers. Of these, the high level of anxiety in our society is perhaps the most worrisome. People have always used alcohol to counter anxiety, and alcohol consumption is on the rise. In addition, we now consume massive quantities of man-made antidepressants. A study of Montreal doctors showed that some of them prescribe antidepressants up to 300 times a month.

Antidepressants are prescribed for people who suffer symptoms such as those experienced by people who are sensitive to lunar phases or to the witches' winds: anxiety, indecision, inexplicable depression, insomnia, irritability, panic attacks.

A number of variables contribute to the harmful concentrations of pos-ions that pollute our indoor environments.

Insulation

We take great pains to insulate the buildings we live and work in against variations of outside temperature, both to save money and to reduce energy consumption.

Soyka cites the interesting example of the Rothschild Bank in Paris (Soyka 81). One day, looking for a department in the bank's splendid new building, Soyka was told that the department had moved back to the old location. Once there, he asked about the reasons for the return. He was told that in the new building, the personnel had caught colds and felt poorly all the time. Because the department did not have to be in the new building to carry out its business, it had reclaimed its old offices, even though the facilities there were dated. People who had complained of listlessness, depression and headaches quickly felt well again.

At the end of the 1997-1998 school year, the authorities of a Toronto-area school board noticed that two of the commission's schools had posted noticeably low professor and student absentee rates. Grades in both schools had also improved significantly over previous years. The board wanted to know what new initiatives could account for the statistical anomaly. The only change was that both schools had installed two ionizers in every classroom at the beginning of the school year. In 1998-1999, the school board decided to put ionizers in all its classrooms.

Those who have had children in daycare surely remember the frightening number of diseases young children are likely to catch in a year. In our northern regions, diseases are most frequent when the temperature cools down and heating systems are turned on. Not knowing better, I once provided one of my daughters' classrooms with a humidifier. Today, I would also install an ionizer in order to prevent the transmission of airborne bacteria and thus reduce the risk of contamination.

Chemicals and aerosols

Pasteur taught us that microorganisms are living beings that reproduce and are propagated. The 20th century has taken information very seriously and invented countless products to prevent the propagation of microbes. Every day, we use liquid and aerosol detergents to clean floors, bathrooms, dishes and furniture. The particles released by these chemical detergent aerosols accumulate in buildings that recirculate air. No larger than .05 to 5 microns, they are light enough to float in the air and be inhaled. Ironically, the air we breathe is increasingly polluted by our search for cleanliness. In fact, the air inside a typical North American home is considered to be four times more polluted than that outside. Perhaps this explains why the rate of pulmonary diseases among women, who spend more time inside than out, has increased by 80% over the last decade

Electric and electronic appliances

Almost all households have electric appliances such as stoves, toasters, heating systems, microwave ovens, sound systems, television sets and computers. All of these contribute to our modern comfort, but also create magnetic fields and produce pos-ions. A television or computer screen produces one million pos-ions a minute. Because the concentration is strongest near the source of transmission, computers, which are always at arms' length, pose greater risks than televisions, which we watch from a distance.

The Standard Bank of South Africa housed its data processing department in basement rooms. Ninety-one operators worked there, using computers and other electronic instruments to process $200 million in cheques per day. Tension was so high and depression so widespread that the managers installed ionizers, acting out of despair rather than conviction. Two years later, a management representative reported that the ionizers had improved the work environment, noting that the rate of error among operators had dropped from 2.5% to 0.5%. Another bank in Johannesburg imitated the Standard Bank and obtained similar results in its computer rooms.

In Norway, Olsen studied the electric environment of people who work in front of computer screens (Robert 71). In normal air, a person receives a positive charge of 3 volts; at 45 cm from a cathode-ray tube, the positive charge is 150 volts, that is to say fifty times higher. Unfortunately, this positive charge attracts neg-ions to the screen and propels pos-ions toward the operator at a rate of one million positive charges per cubic centimeter per minute.

To improve the quality of life and productivity of computer operators, one should therefore install a sufficient quantity of ionizers in their work space. My office, which has a surface area of some ten square meters, is equipped with two ionizers, each of which generates one trillion neg-ions a second. The positive bands of these ionizers attract dirt, and although no one in the office smokes, they are frighteningly filthy after just a short time.

Synthetic materials

When we walk on synthetic carpets, we sometimes accumulate static electricity because of the friction caused by our shoes. Aerosol furniture polishes also produce static electricity, as do clothes made of untreated synthetic material.

Mr. Bach, director of the Danish Air Ionization Institute, worked in several hospitals to treat victims of asthma and respiratory diseases (Soyka 119). He reported the case of a woman who suffered from asthma in her own home, but not in those of certain friends. When the installation of an ionizer provided no relief, Bach studied her apartment, comparing it with the houses in which she felt well. Although he discovered that the woman liked synthetic clothing, that fact was not enough to explain her symptoms. He went on to study her house-cleaning habits and discovered that she treated her furniture with a polish containing silicone. Lab tests show that these products, when applied with rags, produce a positive charge. In the homes in which she felt well, furniture was polished with traditional waxes that do not produce electric charges. Bach coated his client's furniture with anti-static products and advised her to buy untreated antiques. The woman complied, and her asthma attacks ceased.

We have all experienced electric shock, perhaps while removing a piece of clothing, brushing against a screen or touching a piece of metal indoors. This can happen even where there are no synthetic carpets because most of our clothes are made of synthetic blends that tend to carry an electric charge. If the charge is positive, it attracts neg-ions, depleting our immediate environment. If the charge is negative, it repels neg-ions, driving them out of our breathing environment and once again depriving us of neg-ions. Dr. Watson, teaching in a London hospital, said that to help asthmatics one might have to change everything in an unhealthy environment: clothing, bed sheets, furniture (Soyka 117). He told Soyka about a girl who, in adolescence, began wearing the nylon underclothes, shirts and stockings dictated by fashion. At the same time, she began having occasional headaches, which soon became permanent. Her doctor attributed her problems to the onset of menstruation. The girl, however, recognized a link between her headaches and the kind of clothing she wore. She radically overhauled her wardrobe, replacing all synthetics with cotton, which does not create electric charges. Her headaches disappeared soon after.

Dentists

Of all medical professionals, dentists are those whose environment is most polluted. In a study reported by Hervé Robert, Verdier points out that dentists work in small rooms and with ventilation that is sometimes defective. "They are constantly exposed to a permanent pollution of 15,000 particles per cubic centimeter made up of viruses, bacteria, pollen, drilling residue, emanations from medication and dust produced by the pulverization of cements. They often accumulate static electricity because of the tools they use and the synthetic smocks they wear" (Robert 81). Dentists must also cope with fatigue, the demands of intense attention and the high-pitched sound produced by ultrasonic instruments. It isn't surprising, therefore, that they suffer headaches, dizziness, poor digestion, irritability and memory loss. Verdier pointed out that many of these symptoms can be relieved by ionizing dental surgery and waiting rooms.

The city

We're well aware of the pollution emitted by the many kinds of industry we have created over the last two centuries. As much as we benefit from their products, we prefer that these industries be kept out of our back yards.

Rush hour is surely one of the most disagreeable aspects of city life. For those who commute to work, whether in Paris, London, Tokyo, Sao Paulo, Mexico City, New York, Los Angeles, Bangkok, Manila, Cairo or any other megalopolis, rush hour is an inescapable nightmare. Exhaust fumes from cars and trucks pollute the outside air. Given that some 300 million pos-ions escape from our bodies with every breath, one can understand why rush hour bus and subway passengers also experience discomfort

The car

When I was a child, the cure for car sickness involved attaching a chain to the frame of the car and letting it drag on the road. Grounded in this way, cars shed the positive charges that normally accumulate due to an effect known as the "Faraday Cage". Because of the friction caused by air streaming along its walls, the car, isolated from the ground, accumulates positive charges. Electric fans, air conditioning and pollution also generate pos-ions. Drivers who are sensitive to pos-ions are affected by this overload, just as some people are affected by the witches' winds. Why do some car drivers become so aggressive when they get behind a steering wheel? Every school of psychology seems to have its own answer: a feeling of power, accumulated frustration and the desire to dominate have all been suggested to account for driver aggression. Given the findings of ion research, however, it seems likely to me that aggression and drowsiness result from sensitivity to the pos-ion overload in cars and from the resulting production of serotonin. A French study, conducted by the Institute of Research on Transport and Safety and the Prost Transport Co., showed that ionizers improve driver alertness over long distances. Robert also notes that "cabin odors are eliminated, and there is a marked improvement in the confined atmosphere of the cabins" (Robert 53).

Chapter 6

Ionization to improve our health and well-being. WHAT TO DO?

I conclude this essay about neg-ions with a table that shows what I would do if I were a Head of State, Municipal Mayor, Minister of Transport, Minister of Health, Minister of the Environment and Well-being or Minister of Education .

Table: Actions to promote the presence of neg-ions in modern life.

Measures	Comments
Public Places	
Plant conifers in urban areas	Not only do these trees provide oxygen, but the friction of the wind on their needles produces neg-ions (Corona effect), maximizing the effect of neg-ions.
Construct a maximum number of fountains, even simple ones. Ensure access to these fountains.	A simple sprinkler pipe directed toward the sky could be installed at turnabouts and road intersections.

Public Buildings	
Build fountains in entrances and rest areas	Same as above.
Place ionizer in rest area and meeting rooms.	More relaxed meetings Eliminates odors

Work place	
Install an ionizer in every office	Improves productivity
Place ionizers and filters in dusty places	Alleviates allergies

Computer rooms	
Install at least one ionizer per terminal to counter-balance the pos-ions produced by screens	Improves concentration, decreases fatigue contributes to good mood.

Public Transport	
Place ionizers in crowded places	Reduces rush-hour aggression and anxiety
Hospitals	
Install ionizers	Minimizes contamination

Daycare centers	
Install ionizers	Minimizes contamination
Schools	
Install ionizers in every classroom	Enhances learning and concentration, especially for children with learning difficulties. Minimizes contamination
Cars and trucks	
Install ionizers	Improves alertness and mood, reduces risk of accident, has a calming effect at rush hour

Houses	
Install ionizers in bedrooms	Improves sleep, provide relief for allergy sufferers, stimulates sex drive
Install ionizers in bathrooms	Eliminates odors and germs
Install ionizers in living rooms	Improves mood
Install fine diffusion head on shower	Generates neg-ions

Imagine that your oven breaks down. In a panic, you buy and install a new heating element, but the oven still doesn't work. Finally, you call an electrician. He checks the fuses, and finds that one is defective. He simply exchanges the fuse, and the oven works. We often seek remedies for the problems of modern life without really finding solutions. Creating an environment that is charged with neg-ions is no more difficult than replacing a fuse. If an ionizer can change something, it is surely cheaper than any other solution we have tried to date.

BIBLIOGRAPHY

Detailed Bibliography (212 references) available on
http ://www.negions.com

ALBRECHTSEN O. – The influence of small atmospheric ions on human well-being and mental performance Intern. J. of Biometeorology 1978-22 (4) p. 249-262.

BAILEY W.H. – Acute exposure of rats to air ions : effects on the regional concentration and utilization of serotonin in brain. Bioelectromagnetics 1987 N° 8 p. 173-181.

BARON R.A. – Effects of negative ions on cognitive performance J. of Applied Psychology 1987 Vol. 72 N° 1 p. 131-137.

BECKMAN Harry L., M.D. - «Negatively Charged Atomic Oxygen and its Impact on Biology and Pathology of Life Processes», Naples, Italy : Proceedings of the Fifth International Congress of Cybernetic Medicine, 1968.

BEN-DOU I. – Effect of negative ionisation of inspired air on the response of asthmetic children to exercice and inhaled histamine. Thorax 1983 N° 38 p. 584-588.

BICHMEIER J. – Der bioklimatische Binfluss Künstilich erzengter atmosphärischer Kleinionen auf das Respirogramm. Elektrokardiogramm und Electroencephalogramm des Menschen – Doctoral Dissertation. Technische Hochshule, München, 1962.

BOUBLIL G.A.D. — Problèmes d'ionisation et d'aéro-ionisation : données physiques et expérimentales. Thèse de Médecine, Paris Pitié-Salpetrière N° 259 1975.

BOYCO A.D., SVERCHKOF A.N. – All Union Conference on Aeroionization in Industrial Hygiene – Nov. 1963.

BROWN G.C. – Geophysical variables and behavior XXXVIII : Effects of ionized air on the performance of a vigilance task Perceptual and motor skills 1987 N° 64 p. 951-962.

BUCKALEV L.W. – Negative air ion effects on human performance and physiological condition. Aviation Space and Env. Medecine, 1984 55 (8) p. 731-732.

CHILES W.D., FOX R.E., RUSH J.H. and STILSON D.W. – Effects of ionized air on decision making and vigilance performance. Wright-Patterson Air Force Base, Ohio Tech. Rep. MRL-TDR, 62-51, May 1962.

DELEANU M. – Air ionization and circunnual fluctuation of anaphylactic sensitivity. Int. J. of Meteorobiology, 1986 30 (1) p. 65-67.

– Influence of aeroionotherapy on some psychiatric symptoms. Int. J. of Biometeorology, 1985 29 (1) p. 91-96.

ENGEL A. and LIESE E. - «Raum inhalationen undersuchungen Kochbrunnen beim Menschen» - Arch. Phys. Ther. 6, 4, 1954.

FRIEDMAN Howard - «Geomagnetic Parameters and Psychiatric Hospital Admissions. Syracuse Veterans Administration Hospital, et al.», Nature Magazine, 1963.

GIANNINNI A.J. – Anxiety states : relationship to atmospheric ca : ions and serotonin. J. Clin. Psychiatry, 1983 44 (7) p. 262-264.

– Reversibility of serotonin irritation syndrome with atmospheric anions. J. Clin. Psychiatry, 1986 Vol. 47 (3) p. 141-143.

GRAEFFE Gunnar et al. – The Ions in the Air in the Sauna, Finland : Department of Physics, Tempere University of Technology, 1974.
GUALTIEROTTI R.– «Stimulation of endocrins glands by negative aero-ionization» Arch. Med. Hydrol. 1964. 24-15.
JORDAN J. et SOKOLOFF B. – Air ionization age and maze learning of rats. J. Gerontol., 1959, 14, 344-348.
KELLOGG E.W – Superoxide involvement in the bacterial effects of negative air ions on staphylococcus albus. Nature Vol. 281 p. 400-401.
KNOLL M., LEONARD G.F. and HIGHBERG P.E. – Human visual reaction time and atmospheric ion density. Report of department of Electrical Engineering Princeton – N.J. Princeton University, 1956.
KORNBLUBH I.H. – Aero-ionotherapy of burns – Bioclimatology, biometeorol. and aero-ionotherapy, 110-112 – Carlo Erna Foundation – Milan, 1968.
– «Polarized Air as an Adjunct in the Treatment of Burns», Philadelphia : North-Eastern Hospital, 1959.
KRUEGER A.P – The effects of air ions on brain levels of serotonin in mice. Int. J. of Biometeorology, 1969 Vol. 13 N° 1 p. 25-38.

KRUEGER A.P. and SMITH R.F. – Anenzymatic basis for the acceleration of ciliary activity by negative air ions – Nature, 1959, 183-1332-1933.
KRUEGER A.P., ANDRIES P.C. et KOTAKA S. – Small air ions : their effects on blood levels of serotonin in terms of modern physical theory – Intern. J. Biometeor. 1968, 12, 225-240.
– Small air ions : their effects on blood levels of serotonine. Int. J. Biometeor., 1969, 13, 25-2.
KRUEGER A.P., KOTAKA S. and REED E.J. and TURNERS S. – The effects of air ions on bacterial an viral pneumonia in mice – Int. J. Biometeor., 1970, 14, 247-250.
METADIER J – L'ionisation de l'air et son utilisation. Ed. Maloine 1978, ISBN 2-224-00434-6.
MINKA A.A. - «Aero-Ionization in Medicine», Journal of the Academy of Medical Sciences, U.S.S.R. Translation distributed by the Office of Technical Services, U.S. Department of Commerce, Washington D.C., 1961.
MORTON L.L. – Negative air ionization improves memory and attention in learning-disabled and mentally retarted children. J. of Abnormal Child Psychology 1984, 12 (2), p. 353-366.

OLIVEREAU J.M – L'ionisation atmosphérique et ses conséquences sur le comportement des animaux et des hommes. Année Psychologique, 1976 N° 76 p. 213-244.
REITER R. – Frequency distribution of positive and negative small air ions concentrations, based on many years recording of two mountain stations located at 740 and 1780 meters. Int. J. of Biometeorology, 1985 29 (3) p. 223-231.
ROBERT Hervé Ionisation Santé Vitalité Éditions Artulen 1991 I .S.B.N. 2-906236-06-03
ROSENBERG Bruce L. - «A Study of Atmospheric Ionization», Atlantic City, New Jersey : National Aviation Facilities Experimental Center, May 1972.
SELBY Miriam and Earl - «Beware the Witch's Wind», National Wildlife Magazine, August-September 1972
SOYKA F., EDMONDS A. – The Ion Effect – Ed. Bantam 1977.
SULMAN F.G. - «Adrenal Medullary Exhaustion from Tropical Winds and Its Management», Israel Journal of Medical Sciences, 1973.
– «Air-Ionometry of Hot, Dry Desert Winds (Sharav) and Treatment with Air Ions of Weather-Sensitive Subjects», International Journal of Biometerology, vol. 18, 1974.

Made in the USA
Middletown, DE
09 February 2022

60898217R00056